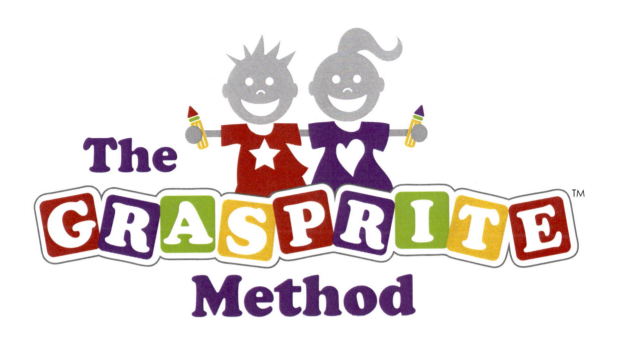

THE **QUICK** AND **EASY** GUIDE TO HELPING YOUR CHILD DEVELOP THE ESSENTIAL FINE AND GROSS MOTOR SKILLS EVERY ELEMENTARY SCHOOLER NEEDS

Lisa Shooman

Illustrations by
Heather Churchill

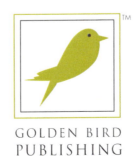

GOLDEN BIRD
PUBLISHING

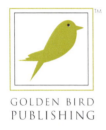

GOLDEN BIRD
PUBLISHING

Published by Golden Bird Publishing, an imprint of GraspRite, LLC
18 Washington Street, Suite 35 | Canton, MA 02021 | U.S.A.
www.grasprite.com

Text copyright © 2012 by Lisa Shooman. All rights reserved.
Illustrations copyright © 2012 by GraspRite, LLC.

ISBN: 9780985629809
Library of Congress Control Number: 2012909030

No part of this book may be reproduced or copied
in any form without written permission from the publisher.
All trademarks are property of GraspRite, LLC.

Printed in the U.S.A.
Bookmasters
30 Amberwood Parkway
Ashland, OH 44805
D10235

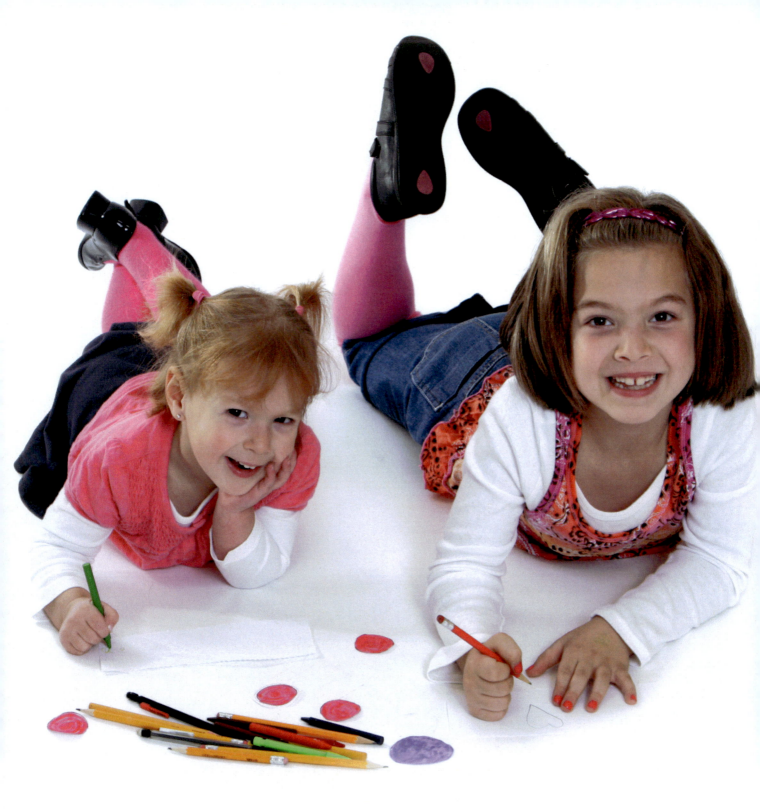

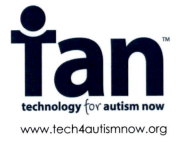

Sales of this book will support Technology for Autism Now (TAN). Technology for Autism Now, Inc. is a 501(c)3 non-profit organization improving the lives of children and families with autism through innovative technology solutions.

www.tech4autismnow.org

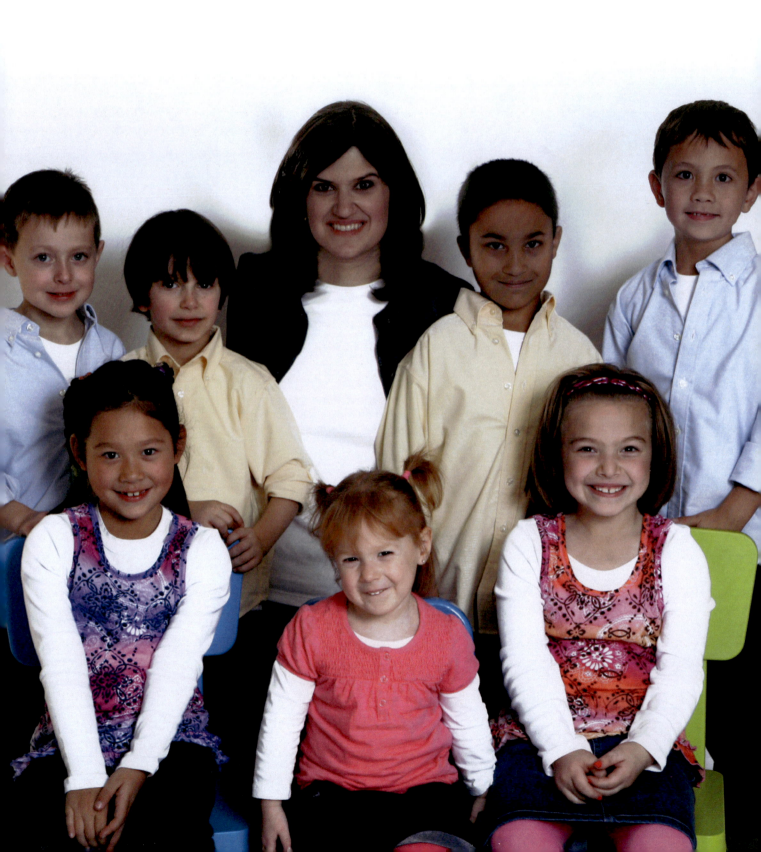

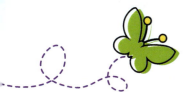

Acknowledgements

Many thanks to my husband, Andy, for his love and support. Thanks to Rachel Stivers and Marsha Schaffel for encouraging me to write this book. Thank you to Kenneth Berman Photography for taking amazing pictures. Thank you to Michelle Winer, MS, PT, pediatric physical therapist and Carol Shriki, PT, pediatric physical therapist, for your professional guidance. Thank you to Debbie Ellenbogen, Margi Rossetti, Evelyn Roth, and Dena Zyroff for helping to steer my boat on the right course. Thanks to the GraspRite kids: Bella, Elianna, Elie, Hanna, Luke, Tavin, and Timmy. You were so fun to work with. Thank you to Lauren Ziskind who came from the heavens and lifted me out of the dip. Heather Churchill, I'm happy the forces brought us together; you are so talented. To all "my children" and my entire family: I owe you so much. Thank you.

Lisa Shorn MS, OTR/L, BSS, CLVT

Welcome to the GraspRite™ Method

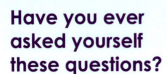

Have you ever asked yourself these questions?

Is my child strong and coordinated enough?

Can my child hold a pencil properly?

Are my child's motor skills age-appropriate or delayed?

Is my child ready for Kindergarten or 1st grade?

You might have noticed that your son or daughter is having trouble holding a pencil, sitting up in a chair, writing, or drawing. Maybe his or her teacher has mentioned that she is concerned because she thinks your child is not at grade level.

When children do not have good core strength and display low muscle tone, they may have trouble sitting on the floor during circle time or they may end up leaning on their desk or table for support. When children do not have good fine motor skills and hand-eye coordination, they will not be able to manipulate crayons and pencils for writing and drawing. When children are not able to process information accurately, they will have trouble with motor planning on the playground and, as they get older, learning in school. [10]

What can you do? The GraspRite Method was created for you, as a playful guide to the most important fine and gross motor exercises for children. Children need to exercise their bodies in a way that's effective and enjoyable. These exercises were carefully selected from hundreds of activities to make the best use of your time. Research shows that these fun movements can help your child improve with the most important foundational skills. The sooner this program is started, the earlier your child will master the exercise program, and the quicker you will see an improvement in his or her strength and coordination.

Adults can benefit from these exercises, too. Get down on the floor with your child and try to do the Airplane Arms exercise or the Kool Kicks exercise with your legs. You will feel your back and trunk muscles working. When you exercise with your child, you can motivate each other, tone your own body, and enjoy spending time together.

The exercises are organized from A to Z, with at least one exercise for each letter, which should give you an easy way to remember each exercise. This book was also designed with the developing young reader in mind. The names of the exercises use alliteration to highlight each letter and emphasize its sound to help with phonics and letter recognition.

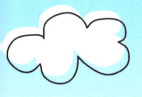

Motor Skills
MYTHS & FACTS

Myth:
Children will outgrow fine motor problems on their own if given more time.

Fact:
Typically, children with fine motor issues need the help and guidance of adults along with a consistent exercise program.

Myth:
If a child displays strength in his legs and arms, he will also have strength in his hands.

Fact:
A person can be strong in one area, for instance be able to lift heavy weights, but still not have good strength and coordination with his hands.

Myth:
You need fancy, expensive toys to help your child improve his motor skills.

Fact:
Everyday objects as show in this program, can be used to help a child develop foundational skills.

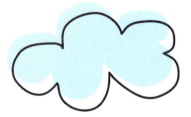

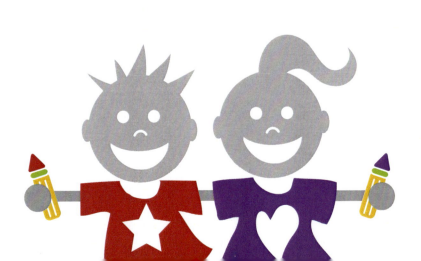

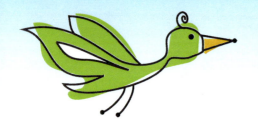 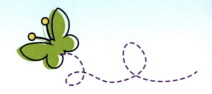

Common Questions

How do I find the time to do the exercises?

GraspRite activities and exercises can be incorporated into your daily schedule. For example, ask your child to do Wheelbarrow Walking with you on his way from the bathroom to his bedroom each night before bed. Bring putty along on car trips and practice making Bitty Balls, Handling Hamburgers, and Pinching and Pulling Putty. Have your child use Clothespin Clamps to hang artwork on a clothes line at home. Do the finger stretching exercises such as Grabbing Grass and Munching Mouths while waiting in line at the grocery store. Take breaks during longer activities and do the Yodeling Yawn activity or practice the Squeezing and Spraying activity in the bathtub.

The American Academy of Pediatrics recommends that children get one hour of physical exercise each day. [1] Some examples of aerobic exercises are walking, running, swimming, and playing sports. Exercise is important for health, learning, and memory. [18] Keep in mind that exercise is cumulative, so if your child rides his bike for 15 minutes and then goes on a hike with you for another 45 minutes, that would meet his daily requirement for fitness.

The GraspRite exercises can strengthen your child's muscles and bones, increase his coordination, and boost his metabolism. Ideally, you should do the GraspRite exercises two to three times a week. When you read this book with your child and you do the GraspRite exercises together, you have the tools to help your child develop motor skills successfully.

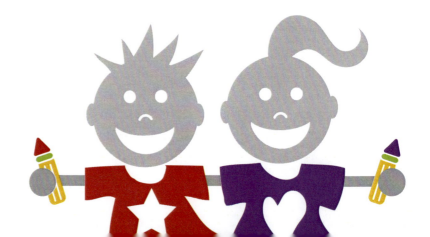

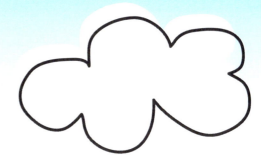

What is Hand Dominance?

When a child favors one hand and he performs better with one hand over another, he is displaying hand dominance or handedness. [14] Calling a child a lefty or a righty is simply saying that he has a dominant hand. Children can be right-handed, left-handed, or ambidextrous. Ambidextrous means that a child is equally skilled at using his right hand or left hand to complete a task. [20] For example, when your child uses his right hand consistently and more precisely than his left hand to eat with a spoon or a fork, then you would say he is right-handed for eating.

Most tasks, like cutting food with a fork and a knife, require the use of two hands. The dominant hand holds the knife in order to cut the food, while the non-dominant hand stabilizes the fork that's been inserted into the food to keep it from moving. When a child consistently uses each hand for a specific job, his hands work more effectively. Children should be encouraged to use two hands when writing or drawing. The dominant hand holds the marker or crayon while the other hand rests on the paper to stabilize it.

How Can I Help My Child Develop Hand Dominance?

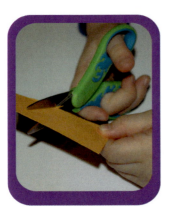

Hand preference is seen as early as age two, but a child may switch hand preference up until age six. [20] Hand dominance should develop organically. We don't want to bias a child toward using a particular hand against her natural tendencies. When we consistently place tools on one side, say by always putting a crayon near the child's right hand, she might feel obligated to use her right hand even though she would do better by using her left hand. Place objects in the middle of your child's body so she can choose which hand she prefers. In this way, you will not be biasing your child. The child in this picture is holding a piece of paper with her non-dominant hand and using her dominant hand to cut with scissors.

In first grade, your child should be using one hand consistently for writing and cutting. If a child has not chosen a dominant hand by age six or so, you may encourage him to use one hand more than the other by placing objects consistently near one hand. A child may use different hands for different tasks, but a child should not switch a dominant hand in the middle of a specific task. For example, if your child writes mostly with his left hand, he should not switch to his right hand during writing. When you see your child switching hands, this may mean that his hand is getting tired. When your child switches hands during the course of a task, encourage your child to do the GraspRite fine motor strengthening and GraspRite fine motor stretching exercises with his preferred hand. You will find these exercises listed in the index.

Supplies

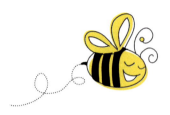

What supplies will we need? If you're like many parents of young children, over-extended and in search of quick but effective solutions, you may prefer to purchase the GraspRite Tool Kit on our website: www.GraspRite.com. The items in the GraspRite Tool Kit conform to all government safety regulations for children's products. You can also make your own kit, as you will already have many of these items in your home, and the others are easily purchased. Gather the items listed below into a clear container and write your child's name on the container. Initially, this will take about 15 to 30 minutes to set up, but there will be no additional preparation time after that.

- 1 small piece of green THERA-PUTTY® (medium) or 1 square of soft clay, which can be found at a toy store or an office supply store
- 1 plastic clothespin, the kind that are used to hold down helium balloons, which can be found at a party store
- 1 small eye dropper, which can be found at a drug store
- 1 small vinyl or rubber ball about 3 inches in circumference
- 1 large ball or balloon the size of a soccer ball
- 6 pennies
- 1 large nut and bolt, which can be found at a hardware store
- 1 shoebox-sized plastic container with a lid, filled ¾ of the way with rice mixed with an assortment of 5-10 small toys like erasers, dice, small action figures, and marbles
- 1 quarter
- 1 regular-size crayon
- 1 spray bottle
- 1 pair of plastic tongs
- 1 toy car remote, real car remote, or carabiner key chain and key

Have fun and use your imagination to play with your child while doing these exercises. Here's to many days of fun and fitness and years of success with your child!

Where should we do the exercises?

All exercises can be done indoors, outdoors, or on the go.

Introduction for Kids

Here are the parts of your hand:

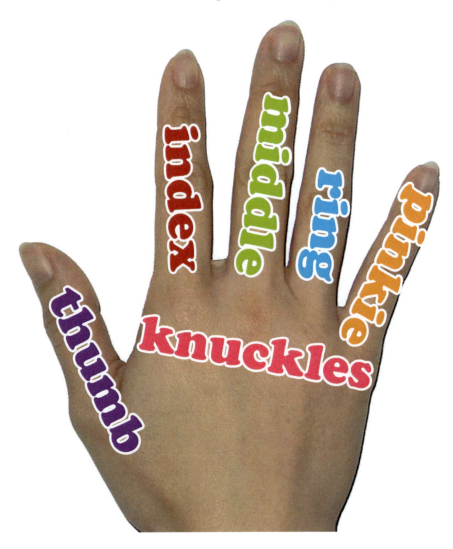

In this book we pretend to be many things,
and we use our arms as if they were wings.

We'll learn movements for each letter from A to Z,
and exciting things will happen, as you'll soon see.

So join with the GraspRite Kids and follow along,
When you move your body, you will become very strong.

A Airplane Arms

1 Hold yourself up on your hands and feet like an airplane taking off.

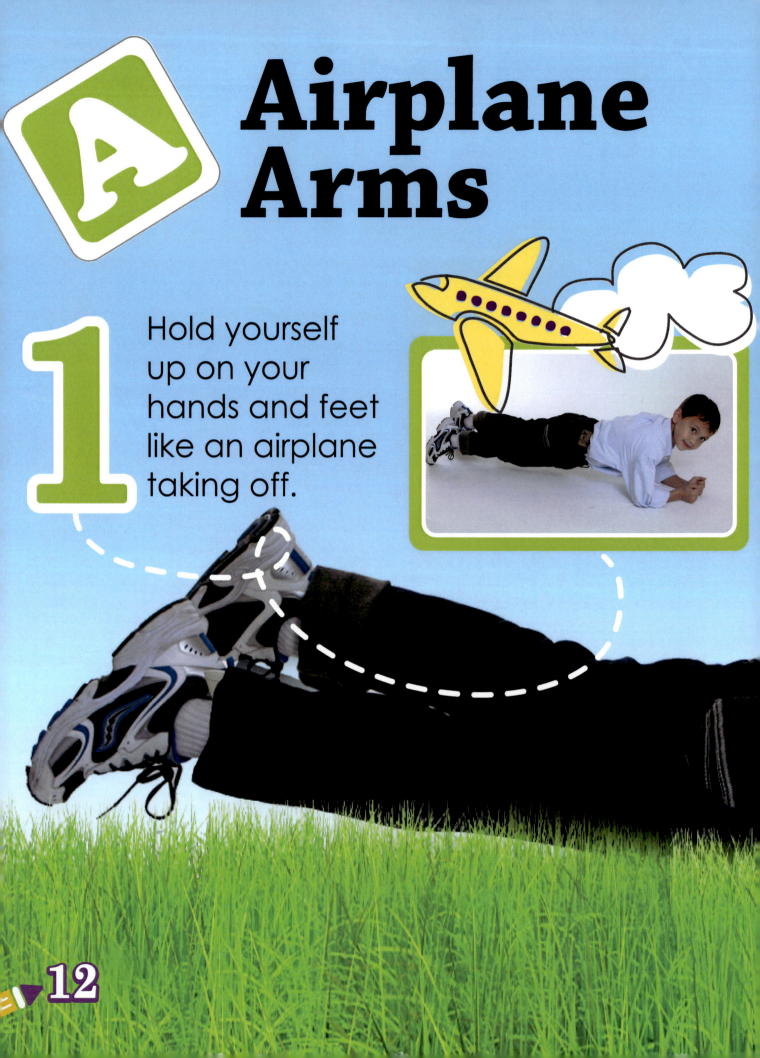

I'm like an airplane that flies in the sky.
I'm like an airplane that flies so high.

2 Then lie on the floor and hold your arms and legs up in the air.

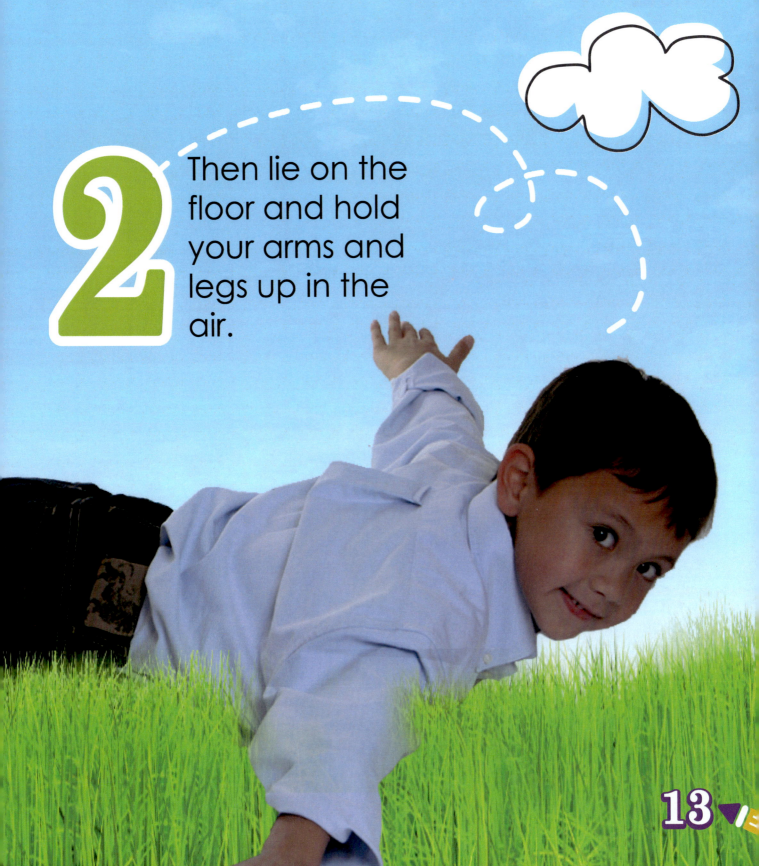

Bitty Balls

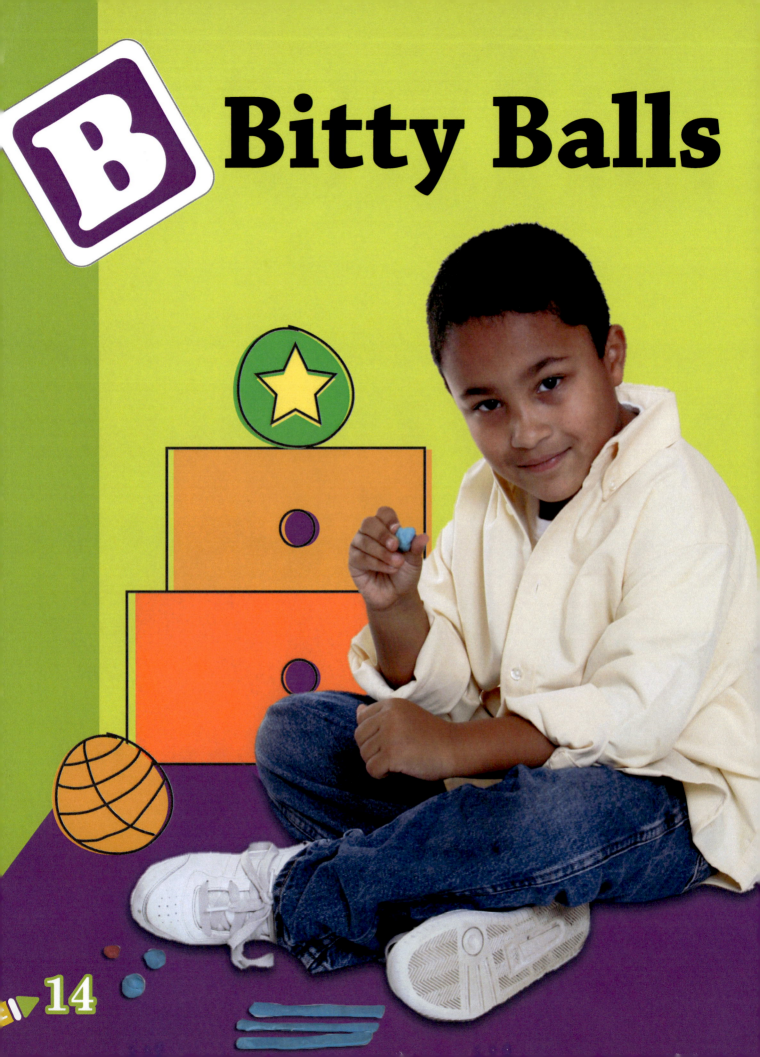

14

Take a piece of putty that is very small. Roll it with your fingers and make a bitty ball.

1 Tuck your ring and pinkie fingers into your hand. Take a small piece of THERA-PUTTY® or clay and roll it into a ball with your thumb, index, and middle fingers. Be sure to keep your fingers rounded.

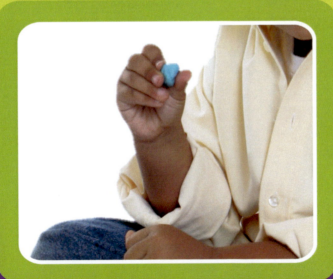

Clothespin Clamps

1 Keep your ring and pinkie fingers tucked into your hand. Make a circle with your thumb, index, and middle fingers and open and close the clothespin.

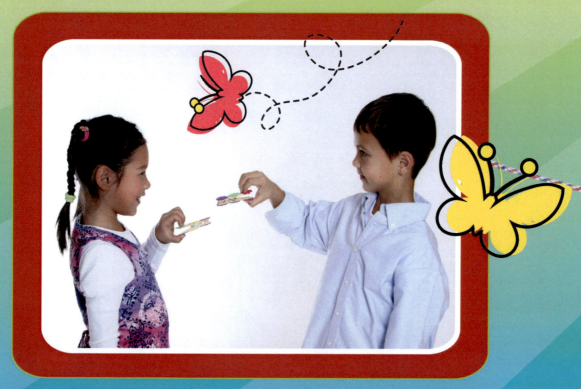

*Please watch your child's fingers to make sure that his fingers stay rounded when doing this activity.

Open and close your clothespin to use it as a clamp. Keep pushing with your fingers -- you're a champ!

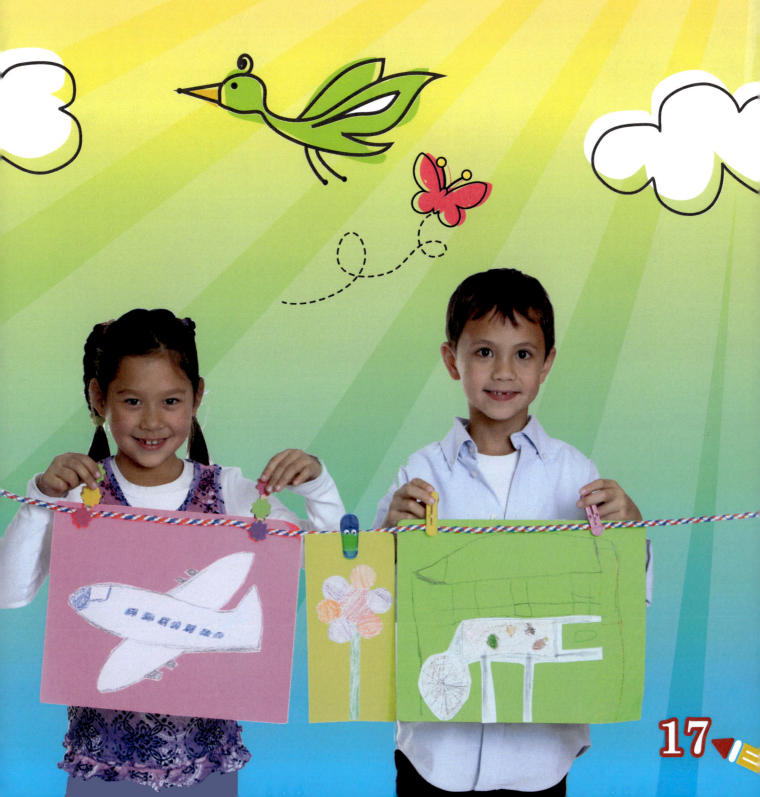

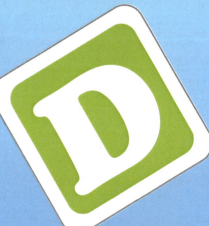

Diving Dolphin

1
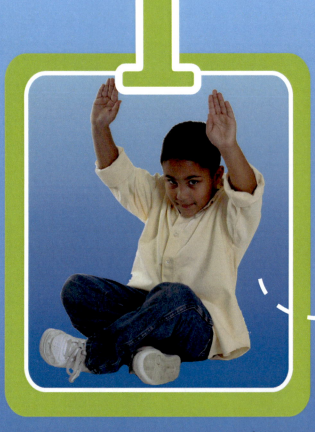

Move your wrists up and down slowly.

2
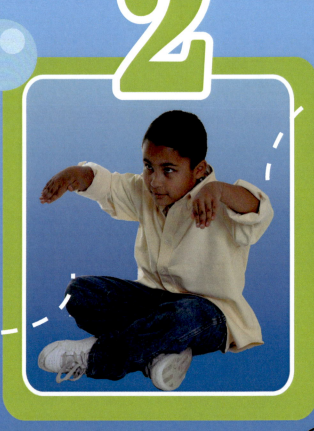

Reach down to the ground

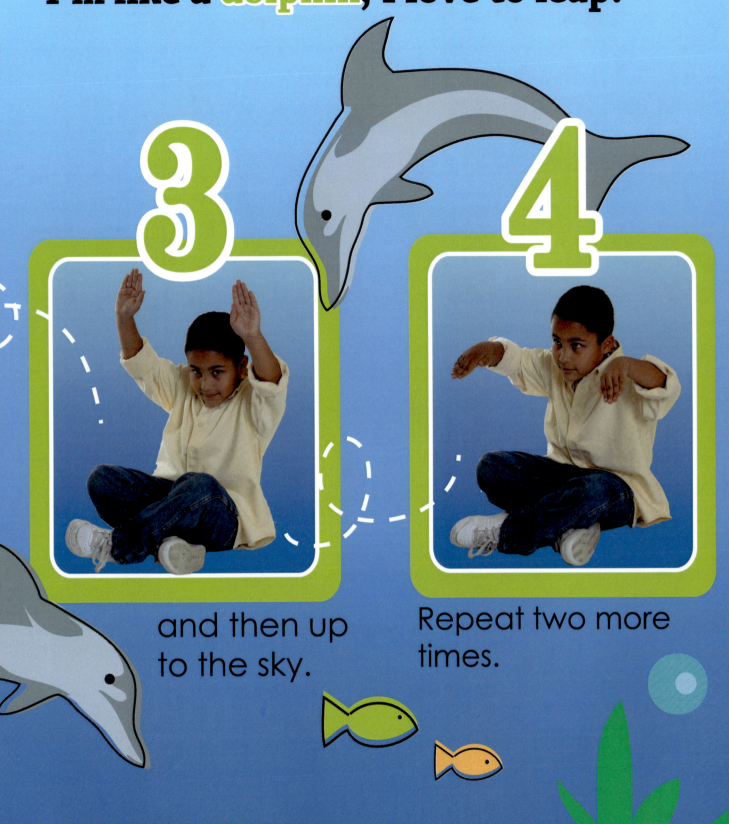

E Eyedroppers

Squeeze an eyedropper with your hand. Join in with children across the land.

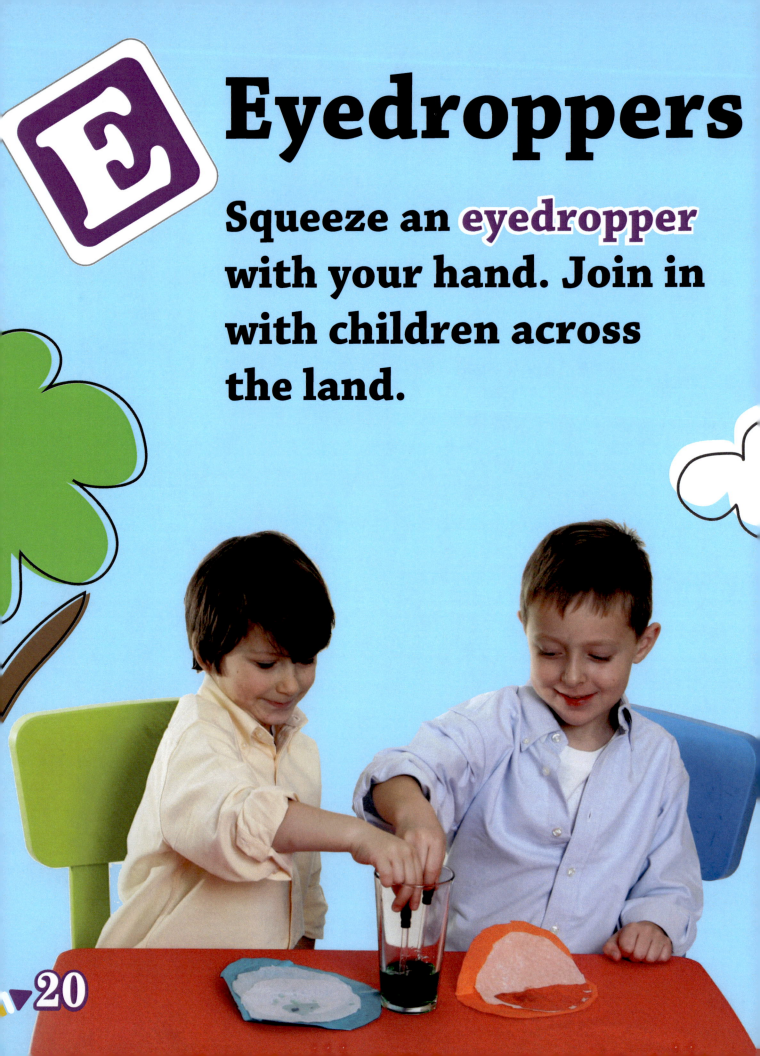

for Everyone

Make a circle with your fingers as you squeeze the top of an eyedropper. Remember to tuck your ring and pinkie fingers into your hand.

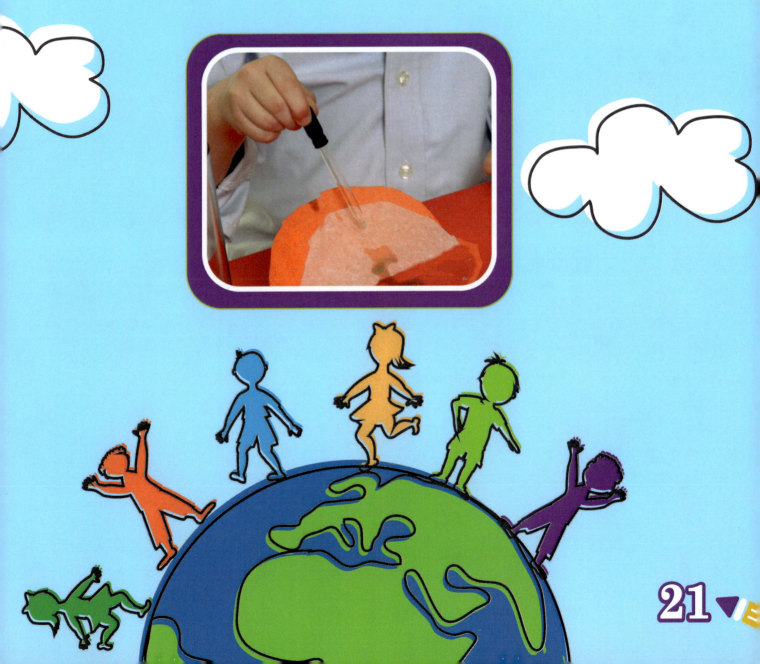

 Flowering Fingers

1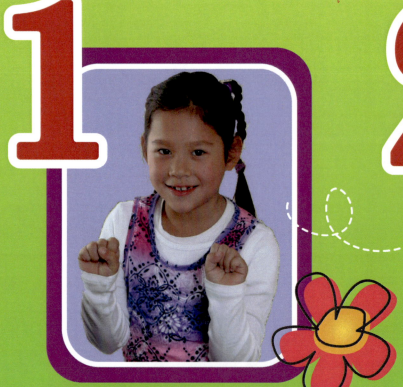

2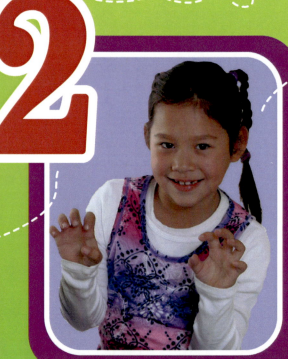

Make a fist with your fingers,

and open them slowly.

Think of a flower with a scent of perfume. I'm like a flower, watch me bloom.

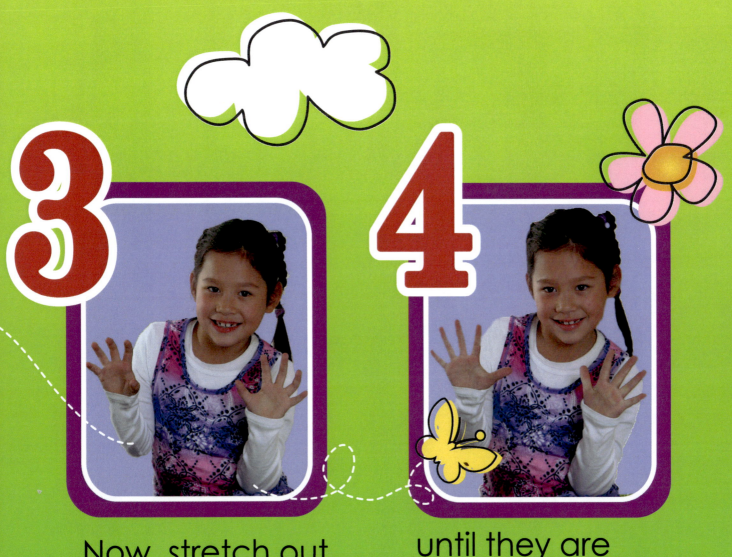

Now, stretch out your fingers until they are completely straight. Repeat this five times.

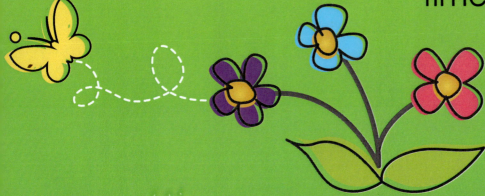

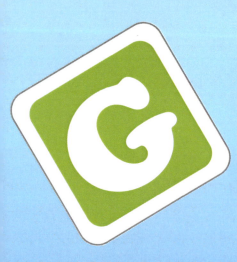

Grabbing Grass

The grass grows in my garden all around me. I want to grab all the green grass I can see.

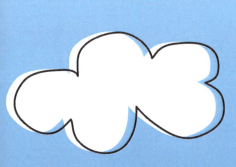

Touch your thumb to each of your other fingers. Go back and forth in both directions. Can you do this with both hands at the same time?

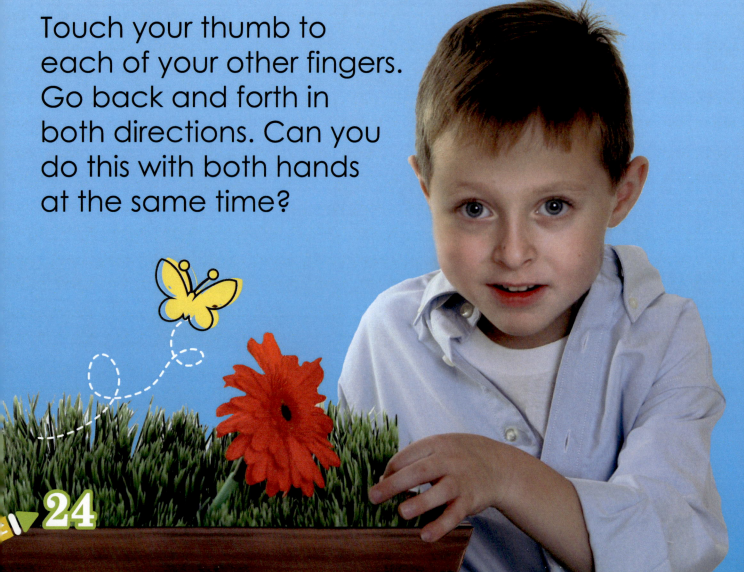

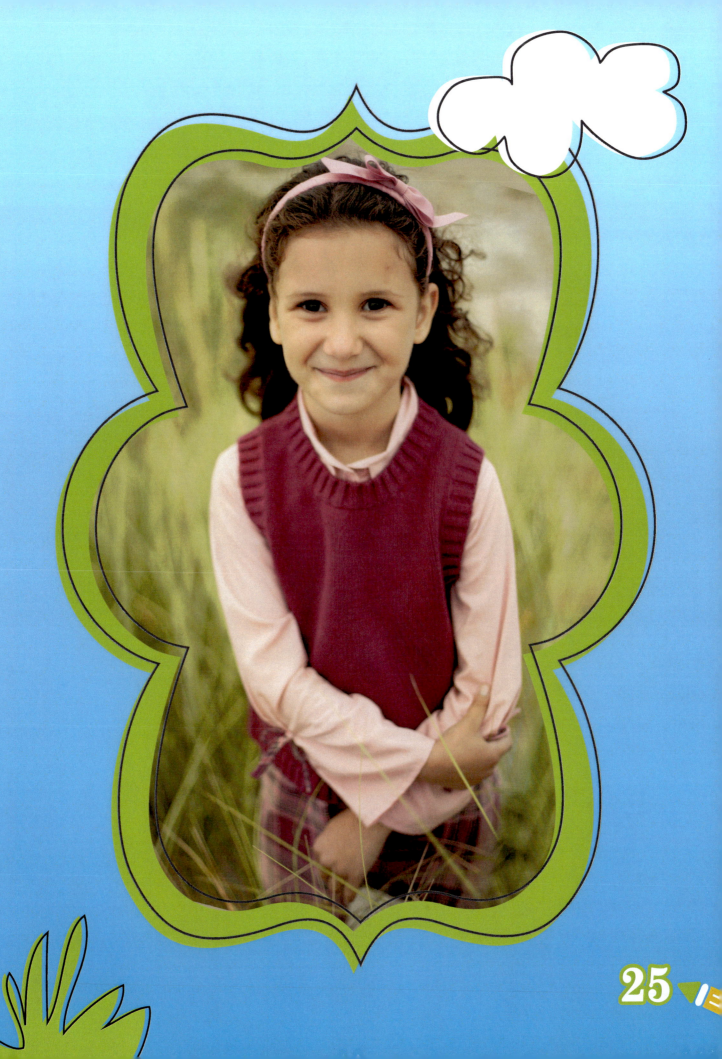

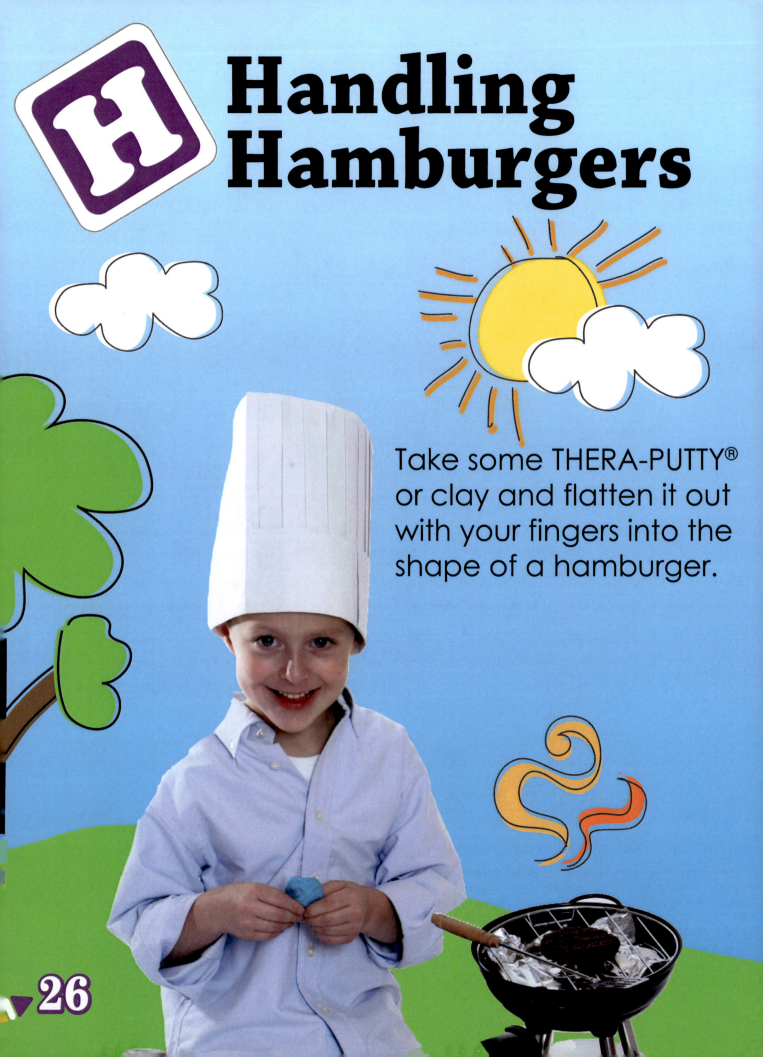

Handling Hamburgers

Take some THERA-PUTTY® or clay and flatten it out with your fingers into the shape of a hamburger.

I'm making a **hamburger** to cook on a grill. I flip it over; oh what a thrill!

1
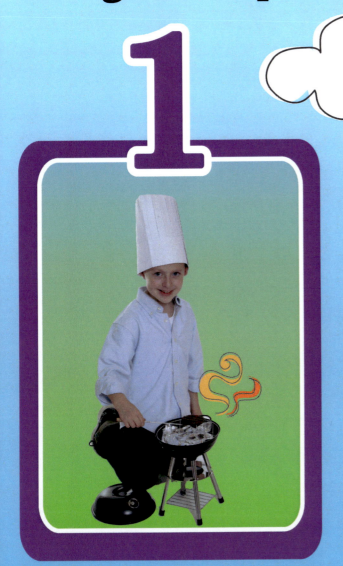

Place a pretend or a real hamburger on a spatula. Hold a spatula in your hand while keeping your palm up.

2
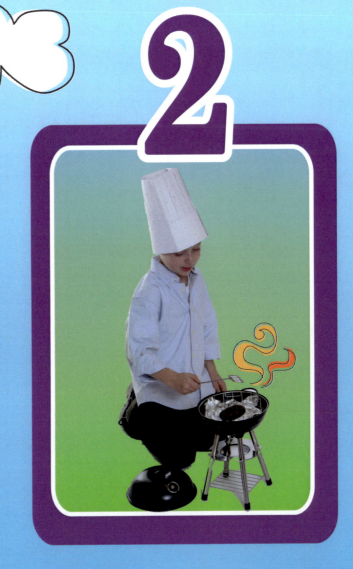

Then, turn your palm down to flip the hamburger over.

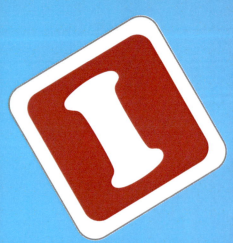

Inching Inchworm

Inch up like an inchworm; curl up to your knee. This is fun, don't you agree?

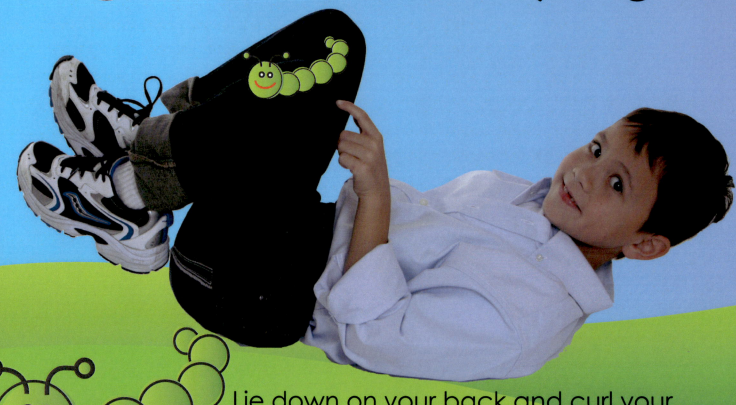

Lie down on your back and curl your body into a ball. Bend your legs and your head towards your chest. While you are curled up, pretend your finger is an inchworm crawling on your knee. Bend only your index finger and keep your other fingers bent in a fist.

Joyful Jumps

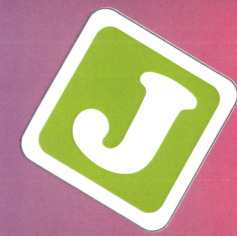

I like to **jump** with my hands in a chair.
I **jump** on one leg, so high in the air.

1
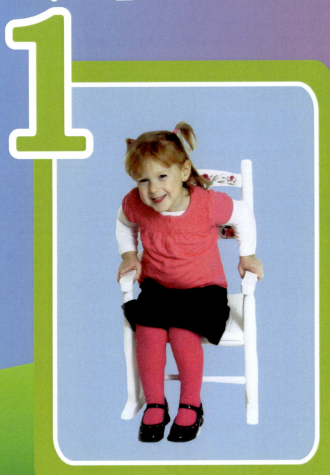

2
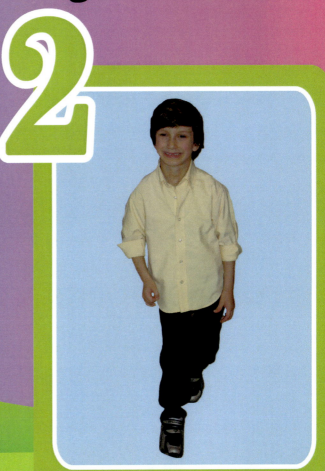

While sitting in a chair, keep your hands flat on the seat or armrests and lift your backside up in the air.

Stand on one leg at a time and jump up and down.

Kool Kicks

Kicking with my finger is such a cool trick. When I'm on my back, watch out for my kick.

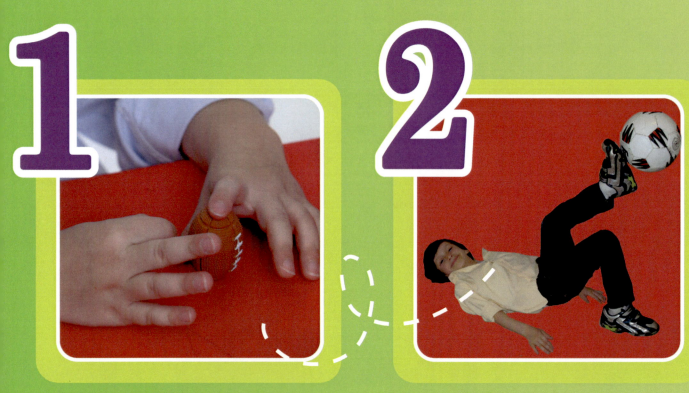

1 Push or flick an object such as a small ball using only your index finger; repeat with your middle finger.

2 Lie on your back and lift your bottom up in the air while keeping your knees bent. Then kick a ball or a balloon with one leg.

Lifting and Lowering

Lift and lower just one penny. Keep adding more and tell me how many.

Pick pennies up off a table using just your thumb and index finger (without sliding them off the table) and tuck them into your fist. Then, place each penny back on the table, one at a time.

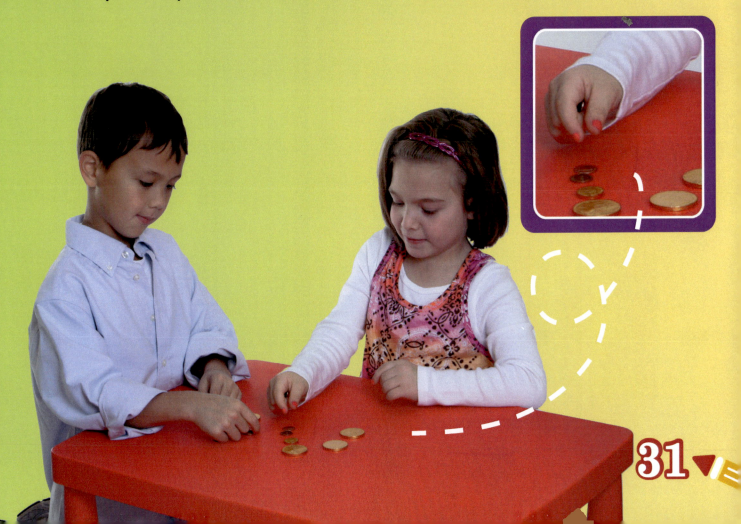

Munching Mouths

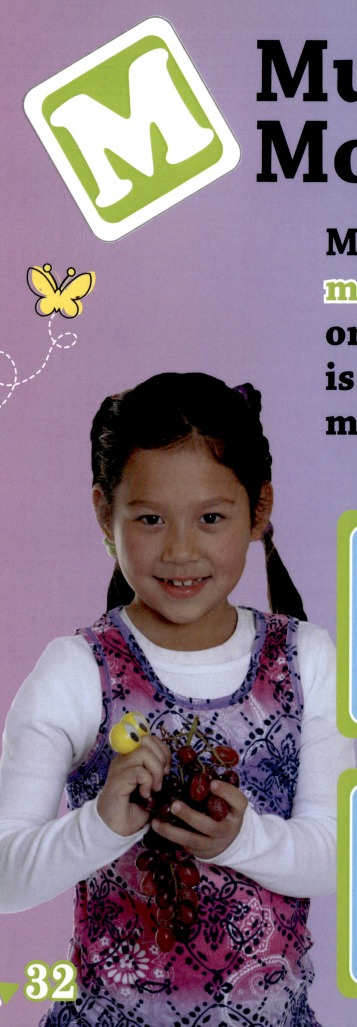

My fingers are like a *mouth*, munching on some grapes. This is so exciting, I'm making finger shapes.

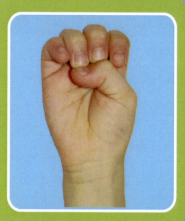

Keep your knuckles straight for this stretch and bend your fingers down.

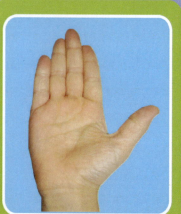

Then straighten your fingers.

Nifty Nuts

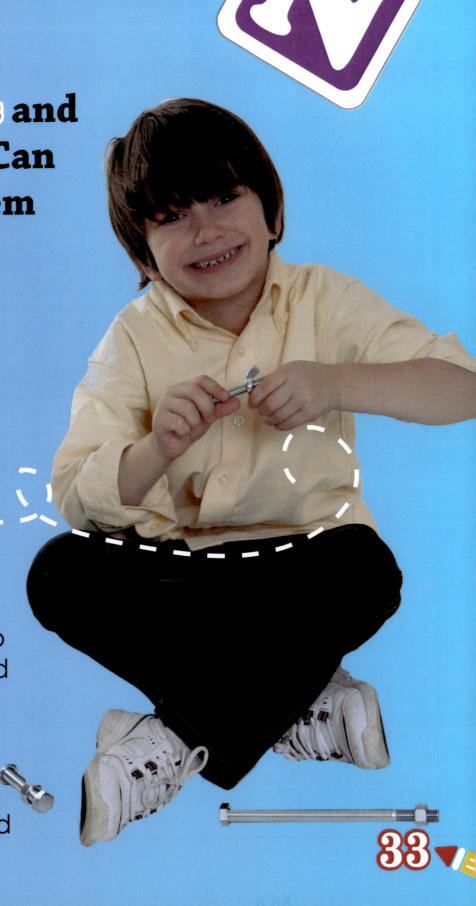

Turning nuts and bolts is fun. Can you twist them one by one?

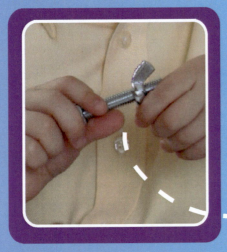

Use both hands to twist a nut up and down a bolt. Keep your ring finger and pinkie bent. Use your thumb and your index finger, then your thumb with your index and middle fingers.

Only Objects

Hide small objects like a pair of dice. Take them out as you find them -- but please leave the rice!

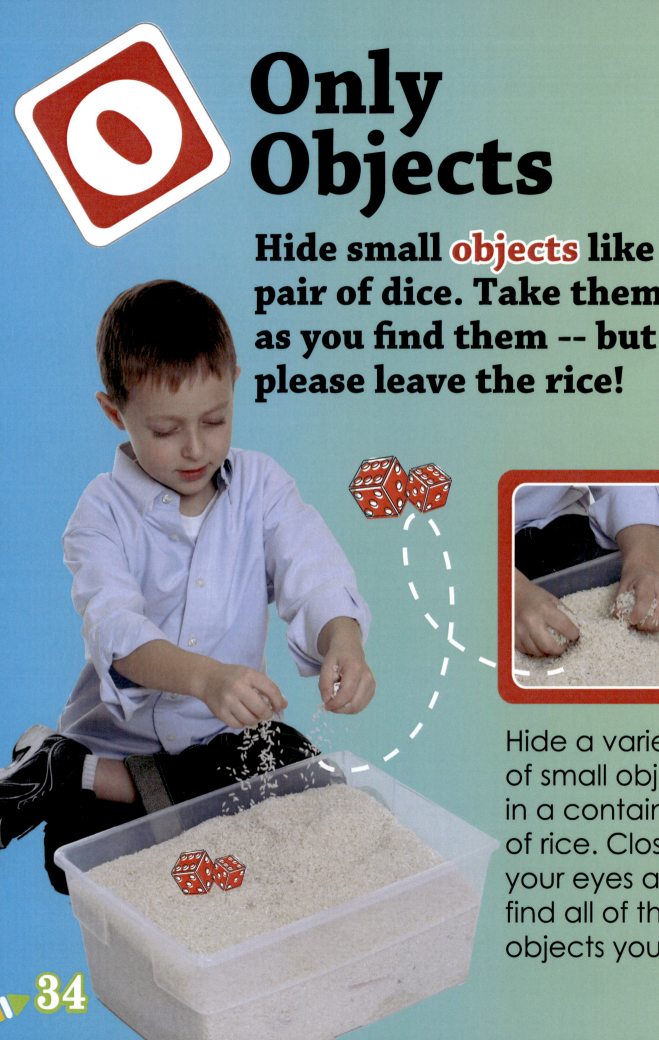

Hide a variety of small objects in a container of rice. Close your eyes and find all of the objects you hid.

Pulling and Pinching Putty

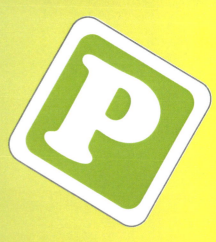

Pull your putty apart.
Then make a work of art.

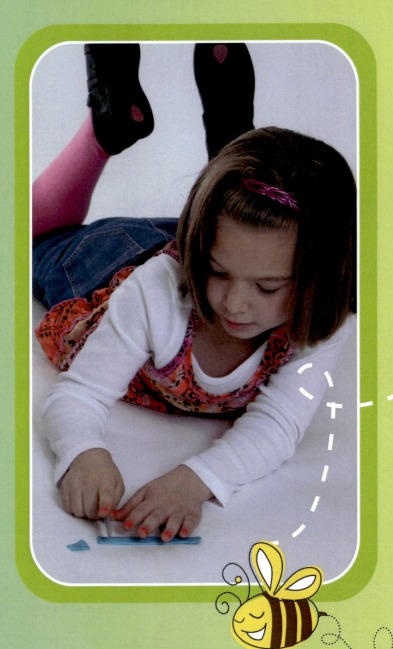

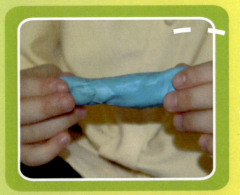

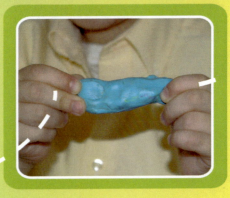

Pull clay or THERA-PUTTY® with your hands. Pinch and pull the putty between your thumb and each finger.

Quick Quarter

I've got a **quarter** that I give a quick flip. Playing with my **quarter** will help me with my grip.

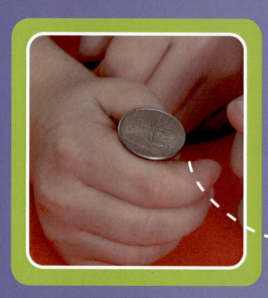

Place a quarter on your thumb and flick the quarter up. Bend your other fingers but don't move them.

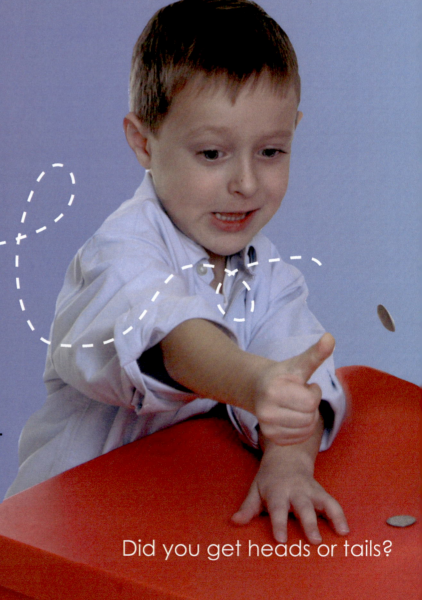

Did you get heads or tails?

Rocking n' Rolling

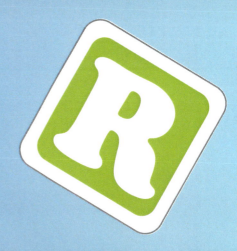

Rock and **roll** a crayon with your hand. Pretend you're playing in a **rock n' roll** band.

1
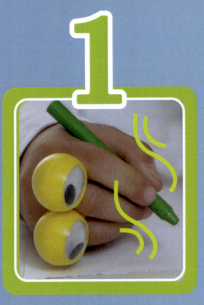

Rock a crayon by holding the crayon with your thumb, index, and middle fingers, then bend and straighten these fingers.

2

Now, roll a crayon with your thumb, index, and middle fingers. Keep your ring finger and pinkie curled into your hand.

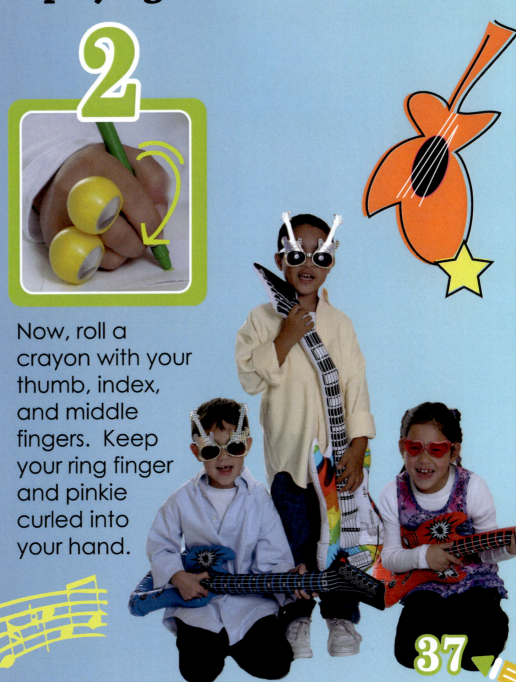

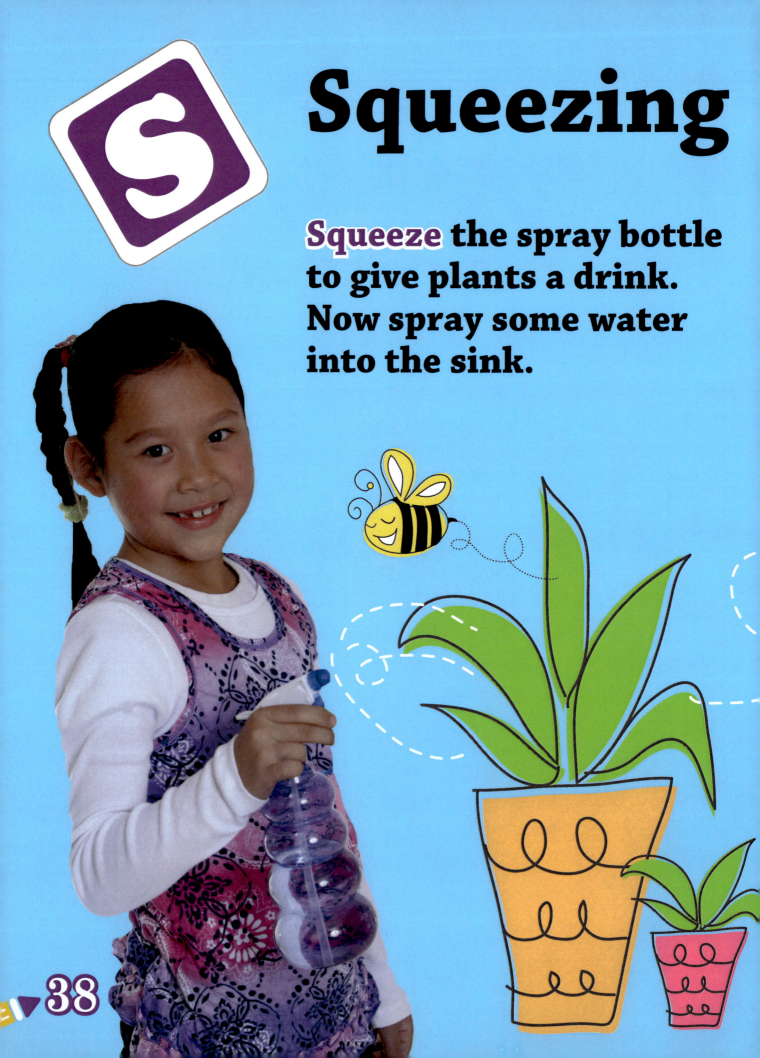

Squeezing

Squeeze the spray bottle to give plants a drink. Now spray some water into the sink.

and Spraying

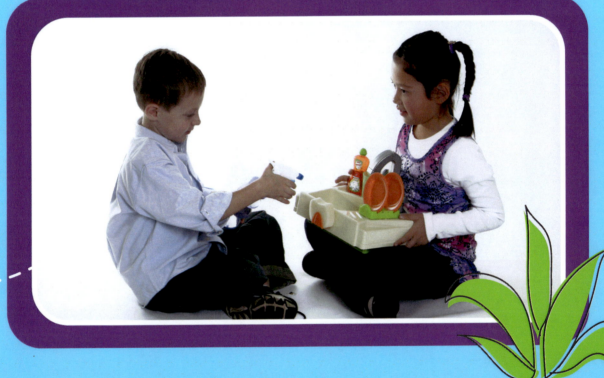

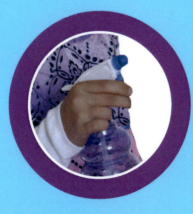 Hold the top part of the spray bottle with your thumb, index, and middle fingers. Use your index and middle fingers to push on the lever. Keep your ring and pinkie fingers bent.

Touching

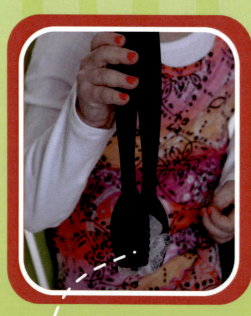

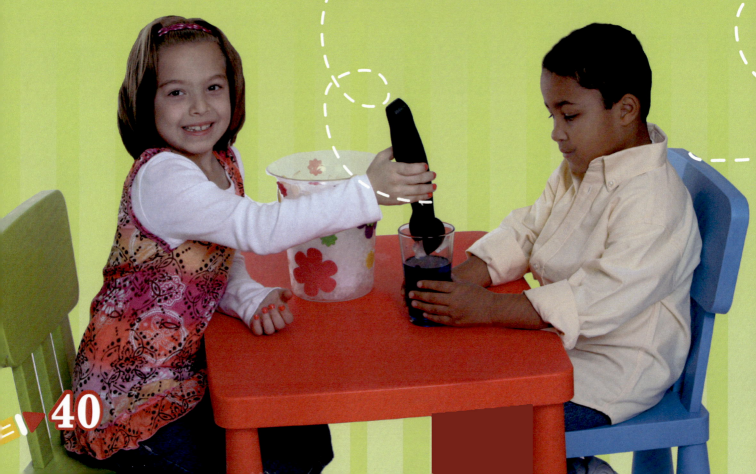

Tongs Together

Press tongs together to pick things up. Use tongs to put ice in your cup.

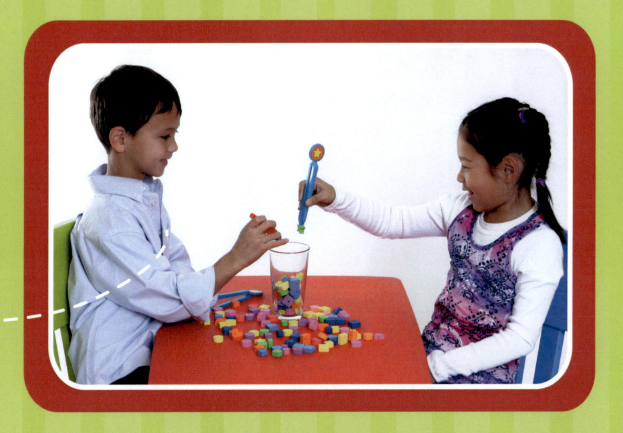

1 Open and close a pair of tongs with your thumb and index finger. Keep your other fingers bent.

Ultimate Unlocking

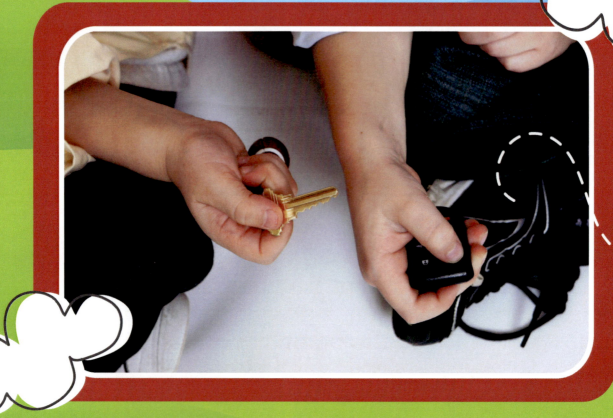

Use your thumb to push on the button of a toy car remote control or real car remote control. Use your thumb, index, and middle fingers to turn a key and open a locked door.

I **unlock** my truck that's parked on the road. Then I drive away carrying a big load.

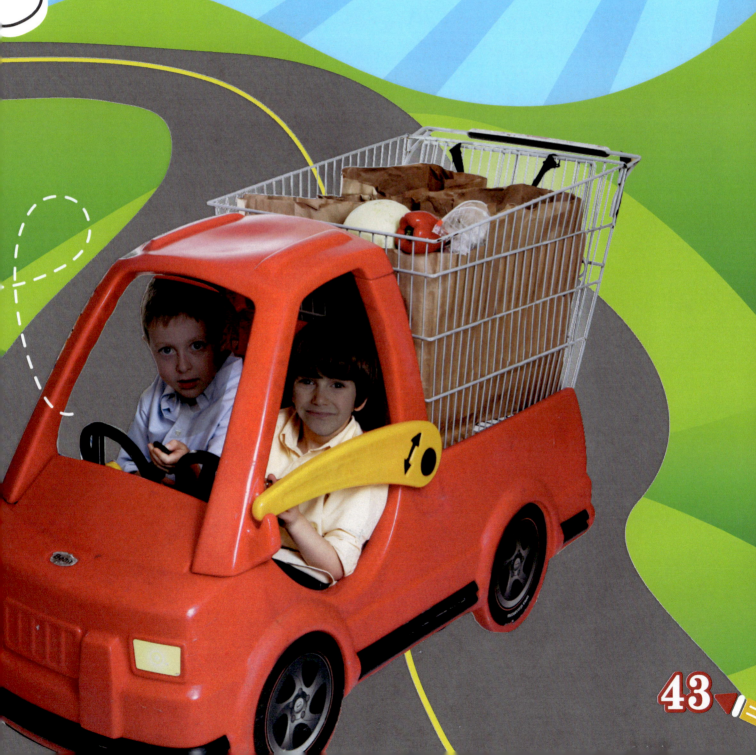

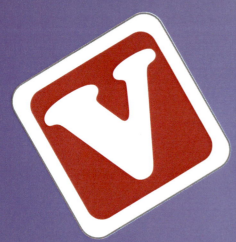

Vibrating Violin

Pick up a pretend violin and make a sound so sweet. Move your arm and play along with the beat.

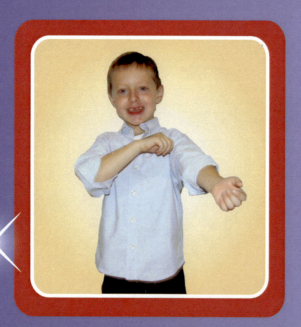

Hold one arm out. Bend the other arm at the elbow towards your chest, then straighten it out.

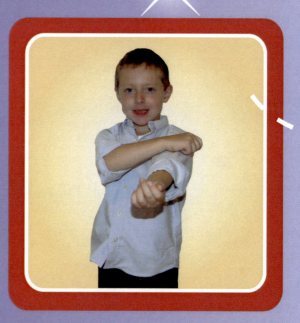

Move your arms back and forth like a violin.

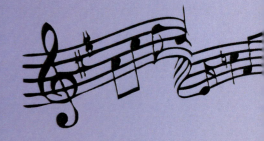

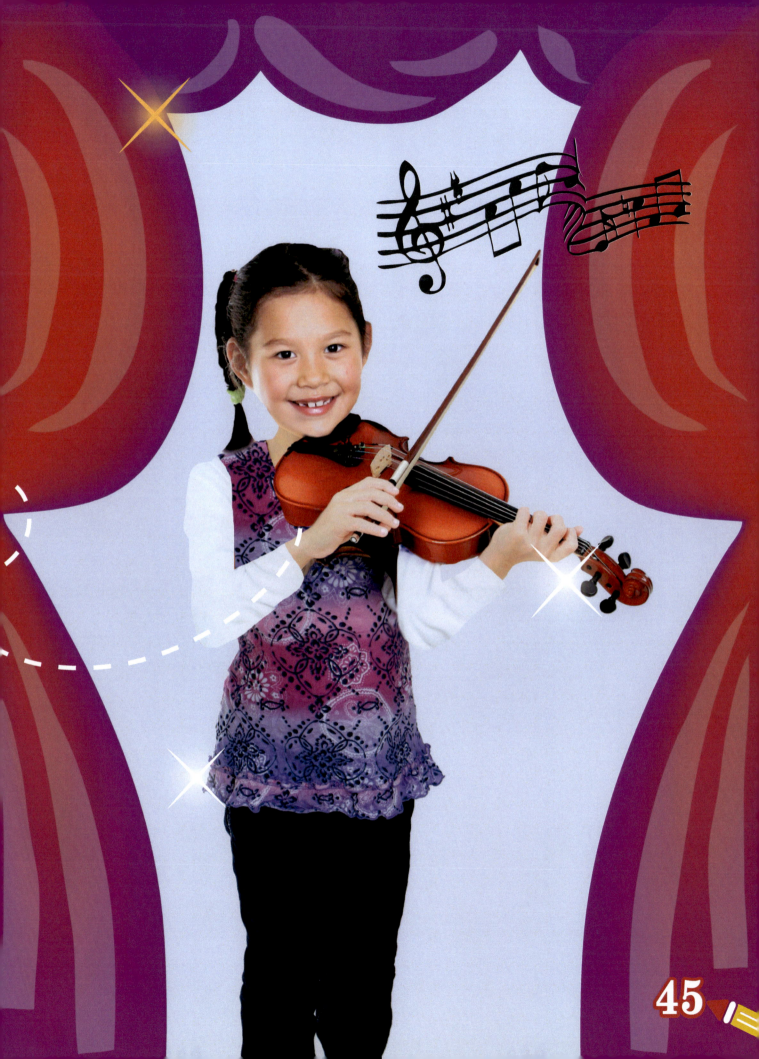

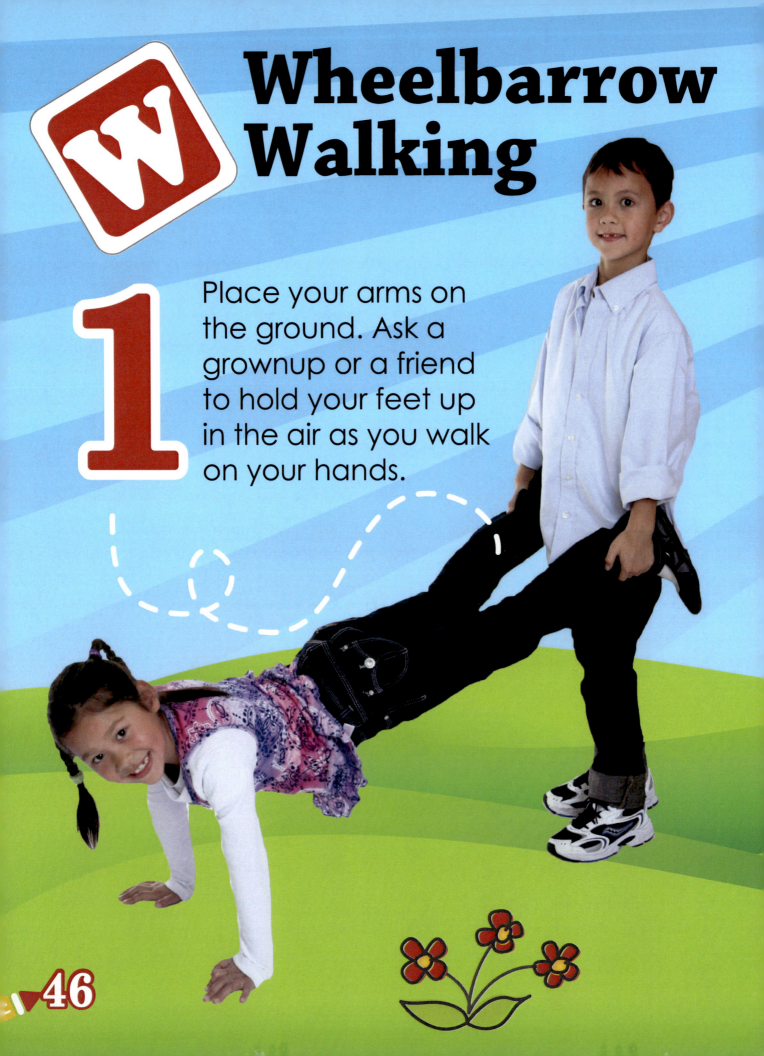

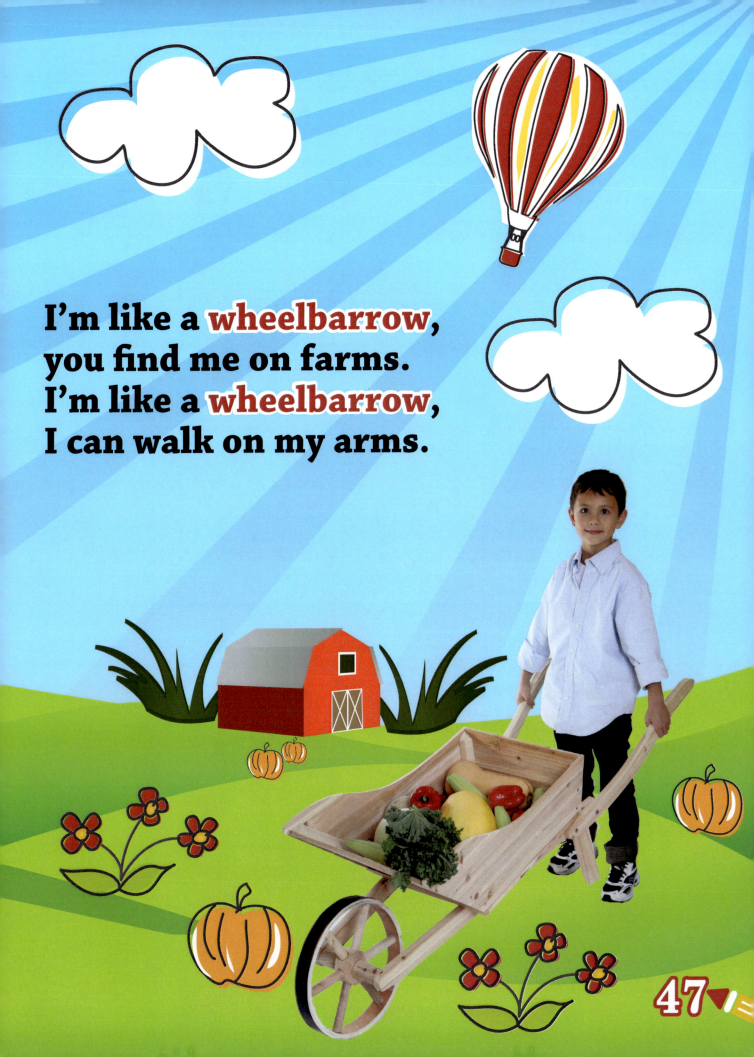

X is for eXercising

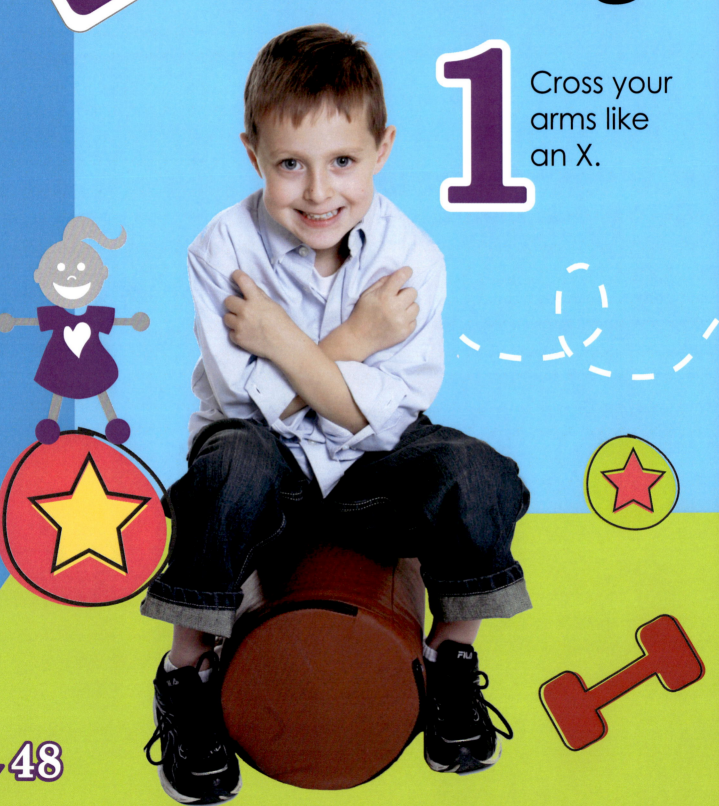

1 Cross your arms like an X.

Reach for a toy, cross your arms like an X. This is so cool, let's see what's next.

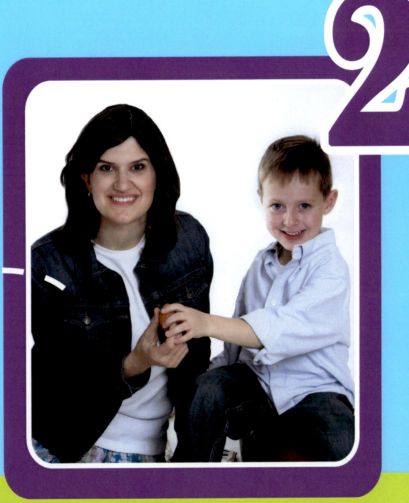

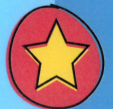

Reach across your chest to the opposite side for an object like a block or a small ball.

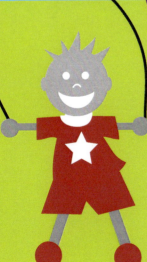

Yodeling Yawn

1
Bend your fingers at the knuckles while keeping the other parts of your fingers straight so that they touch your thumb.

2
Then open and close your fingers for this finger stretch.

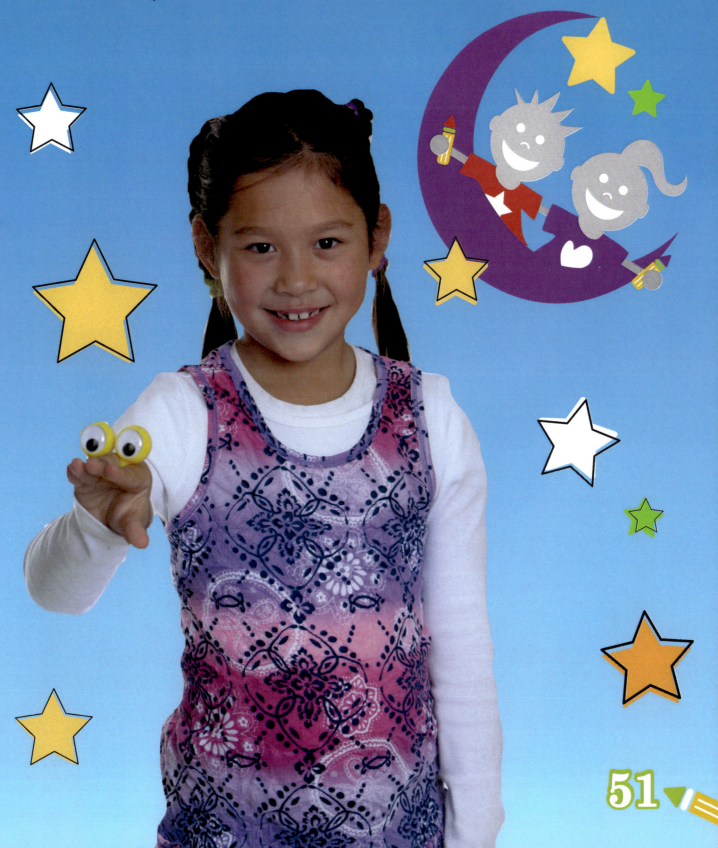

Yawn with your fingers like when you're sleepy at night. Because you worked so hard, you can now GraspRite!

Zig-zags and Zeros

Move your hands in the air to form a zero. You did all these moves—you're my hero!

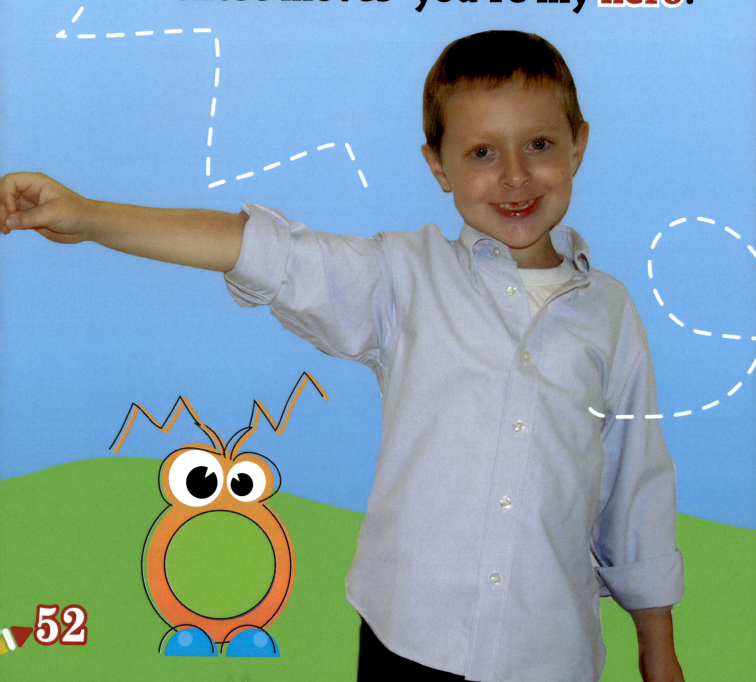

Make a circle with your fingers and pretend to hold a tiny piece of chalk. With your fingers in a circle, hold your arm out while keeping your elbow straight. Then trace zig-zags and zeros in the air.

Fine and Gross Motor Development

When should my child be able to do what?

The GraspRite exercises are typically mastered by ages six or seven but each child is unique and will develop at his or her own pace.[2] Children with autism or other disabilities will take longer to master the GraspRite movements. When it comes to motor and sensory development, girls are typically more advanced than boys. Please use these age ranges as general guidelines only, and don't worry if your child doesn't exactly match these time frames. The benchmarks below should give you a sense of the range of performance that's appropriate for your child's age group.

Your Three-Year-Old

- Your preschooler should be able to start doing all of the exercises listed in this book. Some children may not be ready to do the exercises completely. Ask them to try to copy some of the positions and movements.

- The GraspRite Method exposes your child's hands to objects with different textures and surfaces since his tactile senses are still developing. Your three-year-old child might not be able to smoothly move his fingers around an object, but you can encourage your child to feel objects with his hands. [7]

- You can modify the exercises by using larger objects, or less resistive clay, and by approximating the activities. For example, when doing the Bitty Balls exercise (page 14-15), encourage your child to move his fingers in a circular pattern and pretend to be rolling a clay ball with his fingers.

- Your three-year-old should be able to begin kicking a large ball that is rolled to him. [3]

- It's typical for a child to start out only being able to do an exercise for five seconds, but with patience and practice your child should be able to build up to two to three minutes.

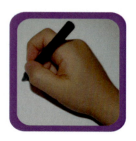

Motor Skill Milestone

At this age, teach your child how to hold a crayon: Tuck his ring and pinkie fingers into his hand and show him how to hold the crayon with his thumb, index, and middle fingers. Let the crayon rest right before the first knuckle. This is known as a traditional pencil grasp. [24]

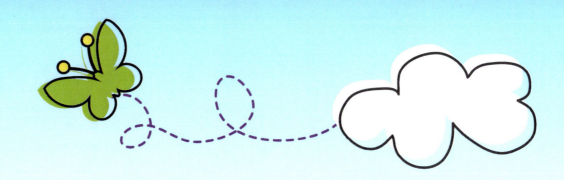

Your Four-Year-Old

- Your older preschooler should be showing signs of improving motor skills while becoming more independent about self-care skills such as dressing, feeding, and washing his body. [7] Some examples of self-care tasks that he should be working on are pulling up pants, putting on socks, and closing fasteners.

- At this age, most children want to do things for themselves anyway, so capitalize on this burst of independence and stand back. Praise your child for all attempts to exert his independence with self-care tasks. Even if your child can't completely finish a self-care task (such as opening food packages), praise him for any part of the task he was able to manage by himself.

- You can begin a task and ask your child to finish it; for instance, push a button half way through a hole and then have him finish buttoning. This gives you the perfect opportunity to praise your child for trying to button his shirt. Each day, "help him" by doing fewer and fewer parts of these tasks until your child is able to manage them all by himself.

- A four and a half year old child should be able to stand on one foot for at least 10 seconds and begin hopping on each foot for at least three hops. [2]

- Encourage your child to hold the Airplane Arms (pages 12-13) and Inching Inchworm (page 28) exercises for about 15 seconds.

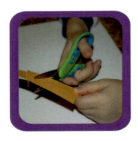

Motor Skill Milestone

At this age, teach your child how to cut with scissors: place her thumb in the smaller hole and her index finger on the outside to guide the scissors. Place her other fingers in the larger hole.

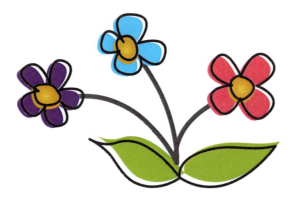

Fine and Gross Motor Development

Your Five-Year-Old

- Your kindergartener should be independently performing all self-care tasks. Encourage him to say things like "I got dressed all by myself," to help foster independence.
- Your five-year-old should be able to snap, button, and zip on his own, but he will still need your help with more elaborate fine motor tasks like thorough tooth brushing and writing.
- Ask your child to close his eyes and feel what you've hidden in a bowl of rice without peeking. Have him guess what the hidden object is without looking. He should be able to feel common household objects and identify them accurately simply by touch. [7]
- At this age, your child should be able to roll a ball of clay in one hand using only his thumb, index, and middle fingers while bending his ring and pinkie fingers.
- The Airplane Arms (pages 12 -13) and Inching Inchworm (page 28) exercises should be held for at least 20 seconds each.
- Your five-year-old child should be able to hop on one foot for 8 to 10 hops without losing balance when doing the Jumping Jumps (page 29) exercise. [2]
- Encourage your child to increase repetitions of each exercise to 10 so he can exercise for about 10 to 15 minutes at a time and build up endurance.

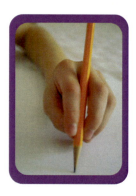

Motor Skill Milestone

At this age, your child should be able to write or draw for at least 15 minutes without difficulties. If your child is only able to write or draw for a couple of minutes or he complains of pain, even if he is using a traditional pencil grasp, then you may encourage him to try a modified pencil grasp. [24] A modified pencil grip is when the child rests the writing tool between the index and middle fingers and then holds the writing tool in a traditional way with his thumb, index, and middle fingers.

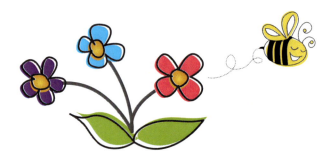

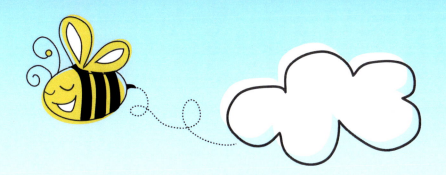

Your Six to Seven-Year-Old

- Your elementary schooler should be able to completely master all the GraspRite exercises and do the entire GraspRite program in about 15-20 minutes.

- Encourage your child to move more slowly through the exercises. When your child moves slowly through an exercise, this creates more gravitational resistance and the exercise becomes harder.

- At this age, because his tactile sense has improved and developed, your child should be able to use his hands to feel around the edges of objects. [7]

- Your child should be able to hop on one leg for at least 20 hops and skip four times with alternating feet. [2]

- Encourage your elementary school child to close his eyes while doing certain GraspRite exercises, such as the Dolphin Dive (pages 18-19) and Vibrating Violin (pages 44-45) exercises, since this can help develop awareness of where his body is in space.

- Ask your child to roll smaller clay balls, squeeze a smaller eyedropper, and use heavier nuts and bolts.

- Gross motor exercise positions during the Airplane Arms (pages 12-13) and Inching Inchworm (page 28) exercises should now be held for about 30 seconds.

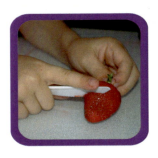

Motor Skill Milestone

At this age, teach your child how to cut food with a plastic knife so she can cut her own food while she eats. Tell your child to stretch her index finger over the top of the plastic knife and rock it back and forth. Have her bend her other fingers to keep them away from the knife. Guide her to hold the food with her non-dominant hand, being careful with those fingers near the knife.

Bibliography

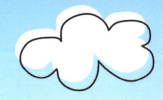

[1] American Academy of Pediatrics. (2006). Policy Statement: Active Healthy Living: Prevention of Childhood Obesity Through Increased Physical Activity. Pediatrics, 117(5):1834-1842.

[2] Beery, K. E., & Beery, & N. A. (2010). Stepping stones age norms from birth to age six. Bloomington: Pearson.

[3] Bernhardt, D. T., & et al. (2001). Strength training by children and adolescents. Pediatrics, 107(6):1470–1472.

[4] Biel, N. & Peske, N. (2009). Raising a sensory smart child. New York: Penguin Books.

[5] Case-Smith, J. (2006). Hand skill development in the context of infant's play: Birth to 2 years. In A. Henderson and C. Pehoski, (Eds.), Hand Function in the Child, (pp. 117–142). St. Louis: Mosby Elsevier.

[6] Case-Smith, J., & O'Brien, J. C. (2010). Occupational therapy for children. St. Louis: Mosby, Inc.

[7] Cermak, J. (2006) Perceptual functions of the hand. In A. Henderson and C. Pehoski, (Eds.), Hand Function in the Child, (pp. 63–88). St. Louis: Mosby Elsevier.

[8] Cohen, L. J. (2001). Playful parenting. New York: Ballantine.

[9] Dennison, P. E., & Dennison, G. E. (1992). Brain gym. California: Educational Kinesthetics.

[10] Dryden, G., & Vos, J. (2001). The learning revolution. Stafford: Network Educational Press Ltd.

[11] Forssberg, H., et al. (1991). Development of human precision grip. I: Basic coordination of force. Experimental Brain Research, 85:451–457.

[12] Greenspan, S., & Wieder, S. (1998). The child with special needs: Encouraging intellectual and emotional growth. Reading: Perseus Books.

[13] Hannaford, C. (2005). Smart moves, why learning is not all in your head. Arlington: Great River Books.

[14] Henderson, A., & Pehoski, C. (2006). Hand function in the child: Foundations for remediation. (2nd ed.). Philadelphia: Mosby, Inc.

[15] Houglum, P., & Bertoti, D. (2011). Brunnstrom's Clinical Kinesiology. Philadelphia: F.A. Davis Company.

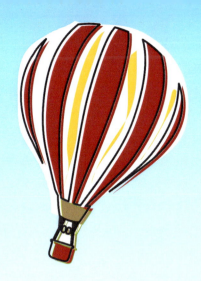

[16] Lefkof, B. M. (1986). Trunk flexion in healthy children aged 3 to 7 years. Physical Therapy, 1(66): 30-44.

[17] Kraus, E.H. (2006). Handedness in children. In A. Henderson and C. Pehoski, (Eds.), Hand Function in the Child, (pp. 161–191). St. Louis: Mosby Elsevier.

[18] Medina, J. (2011). Brain rules for baby: How to raise a happy, smart child from birth through age five. Seattle: Pear Press.

[19] Pediatrics, A. A. O., & Shelov, S. P. (2010). Caring for your baby and young child, birth to age 5. (5th ed.). New York: Bantam.

[20] Pehoski, C. (2006). Object manipulation in infants and children. In A. Henderson and C. Pehoski, (Eds.), Hand Function in the Child, (pp. 143–160). St. Louis: Mosby Elsevier.

[21] Rosenblum, S., & Engel-Yeger, B. (2010). The effects of protracted graphomotor tasks on tripod pinch strength and handwriting performance in children with dysgraphia. Disability and Rehabilitation, 32(21):1749–1757.

[22] Schneck, C. M. & Henderson, A. (1990). Descriptive analysis of the developmental progression of grip positions for pencil and crayon control in non-dysfunctional children. American Journal of Occupational Therapy, 44:893–900.

[23] Schor, E. L. (1999). Caring for your school-age child: Ages 5 to 12. New York: Bantam Books.

[24] Selin, A. S. (2003). Pencil grip: A descriptive model and four empirical studies. Åbo Painosalama Oy: Akademi University Press.

[25] Stilwell, J. M. (1987). The development of manual midline crossing in 2-6 year old children. American Journal of Occupational Therapy, 41(12):783–793.

[26] Wenig, M. (2003). YogaKids: Educating the Whole Child Through Yoga. New York: Stewart, Tabori and Chang.

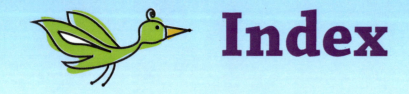

Index

This index categorizes each exercise according to the primary and secondary goals. Some activities target multiple areas. Refer to this index if you want to focus on exercises targeting a specific area.

Crossing Midline Activity
X is for eXercising 48-49

Gross Motor Core Exercises
Airplane Arms 12-13
Inching Inchworm 28
Joyful Jumps 29
Kool Kicks 30
Wheelbarrow Walking 46-47
X is for eXercising 48-49

Gross Motor Leg Exercises
Airplane Arms 12-13
Inching Inchworm 28
Joyful Jumps 29
Kool Kicks 30
Wheelbarrow Walking 46-47

Fine Motor Coordination Activities
Grabbing Grass 24-25
Kool Kicks 30
Lifting and Lowering 31
Nifty Nuts 33
Rocking n' Rolling 37

Fine Motor Strengthening Exercises
Bitty Balls 14-15
Clothespin Clamps 16-17
Eyedroppers for Everyone 20-21
Handling Hamburgers 26-27
Pulling and Pinching Putty 35
Squeezing and Spraying 38-39
Touch Tongs Together 40-41

Fine Motor Stretching
Flowering Fingers 22-23
Munching Mouths 32
Yodeling Yawn 50-51

Forearm Exercises
Handling Hamburgers 26-27
Vibrating Violin 44-45

Shoulder Exercises
Diving Dolphin 18-19
Zig-zags and Zeros 52-53
Joyful Jumps 29
Vibrating Violin 44-45
Wheelbarrow Walking 46-47

Tactile Sensory Activities
Only Objects 34
Pulling and Pinching Putty 35

Thumb Exercises
Quick Quarter 36
Ultimate Unlocking 42-43

Wrist Exercises
Diving Dolphin 18-19
Zig-zags and Zeros 52-53

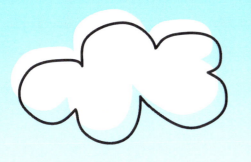
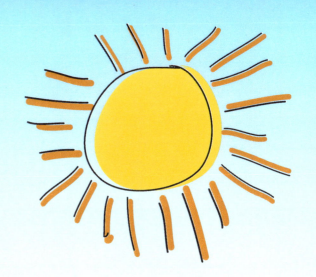

Lisa Shooman, MS, OTR/L, BSS, CLVT

is a practicing occupational therapist, behavior support specialist, and researcher. She overcame a developmental delay as a young child and went on to earn her master's degree in occupational therapy from Columbia University in 1996. Lisa holds specialized certifications in behavioral psychology and low vision.

She has a passion for writing and using her imagination to create fun, educational products for children. Lisa is an experienced mother, and her research includes figuring out how to best guide and nurture her own three unique children.

Don't miss your **FREE BONUS GIFT** found only at: **www.GraspRite.com.** Enter in the code words, **GraspRite Kids**, for free information that complements this book. Please feel free to contact me with questions or feedback via my website.

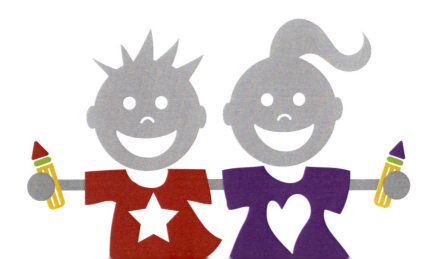
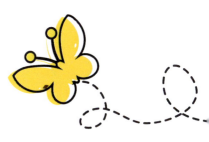

Author's note: If your child experiences pain or discomfort during these exercises, stop immediately. Please check with your child's pediatrician, occupational therapist, and/or physical therapist if you have any concerns about your child beginning or ending this exercise program. It is the adult's responsibility to ensure that the materials for all the exercises and activities are used as intended and conform to all government safety regulations.

Legal Disclaimer: The information contained in this book cannot replace or substitute for the services of trained professionals in any field, including, but not limited to, mental, medical, psychological, or educational fields. Neither Lisa Shooman and GraspRite, LLC, nor their assignees, sponsors, speakers, partners, contractors, or any of their affiliates will be liable for any direct, indirect, consequential, special, exemplary, or other damages to the purchaser or user, including economic loss, that may result from purchase of this book or from the use of, or the inability to use the materials, information, or strategies communicated through this book, even if advised of the possibility of such damages.